I AM WITH YOU

I would like to dedicate this Book to everyone who supported me on my Mental Wellness journey.

My Mother, My Father, My family, My Doctor (Dr.F.Robinson) & My friends. There will never be enough words to explain how God used you guys on my Mental Wellness Journey.

This book is a reflection of the support I had while on a Mental Wellness Journey. The affirmations in this book are short & simple however they are so meaningful to someone on a Mental Wellness Journey. The affirmations are a combination of words spoken to me, words I spoke over myself & words I can only give from my experience of overcoming a Deep Depression. The coloring aspect is a relaxation exercise. I ask all readers to take this affirmation coloring book on a 24 week journey as you are seeking professional help. The book provides 1 affirmation per week to speak, trust, & believe. I hope this book is used as empowerment, inspiration & to seek the presences of God while on your Mental Wellness Journey. If you are reading this page here its not by accident you got a hold to this book. I once was in the same place you are in. Can I share with you God healed me, therapy helped me so much, & my support system encouraged me on My Mental Wellness Journey. God & Therapy is Key to your journey, its a must you are utilizing both. Let this book support you & be a reminder that you are not alone, **I am with You.**

For more information on:
Breaking The Silence Mental Health Foundation & Kenya Adiva
Seek Websites:
www.BreakTheSilenceMentalHealth.com
www.KenyaAdiva.com

Believe
YOU CAN
& YOU
will

You Are Brave!

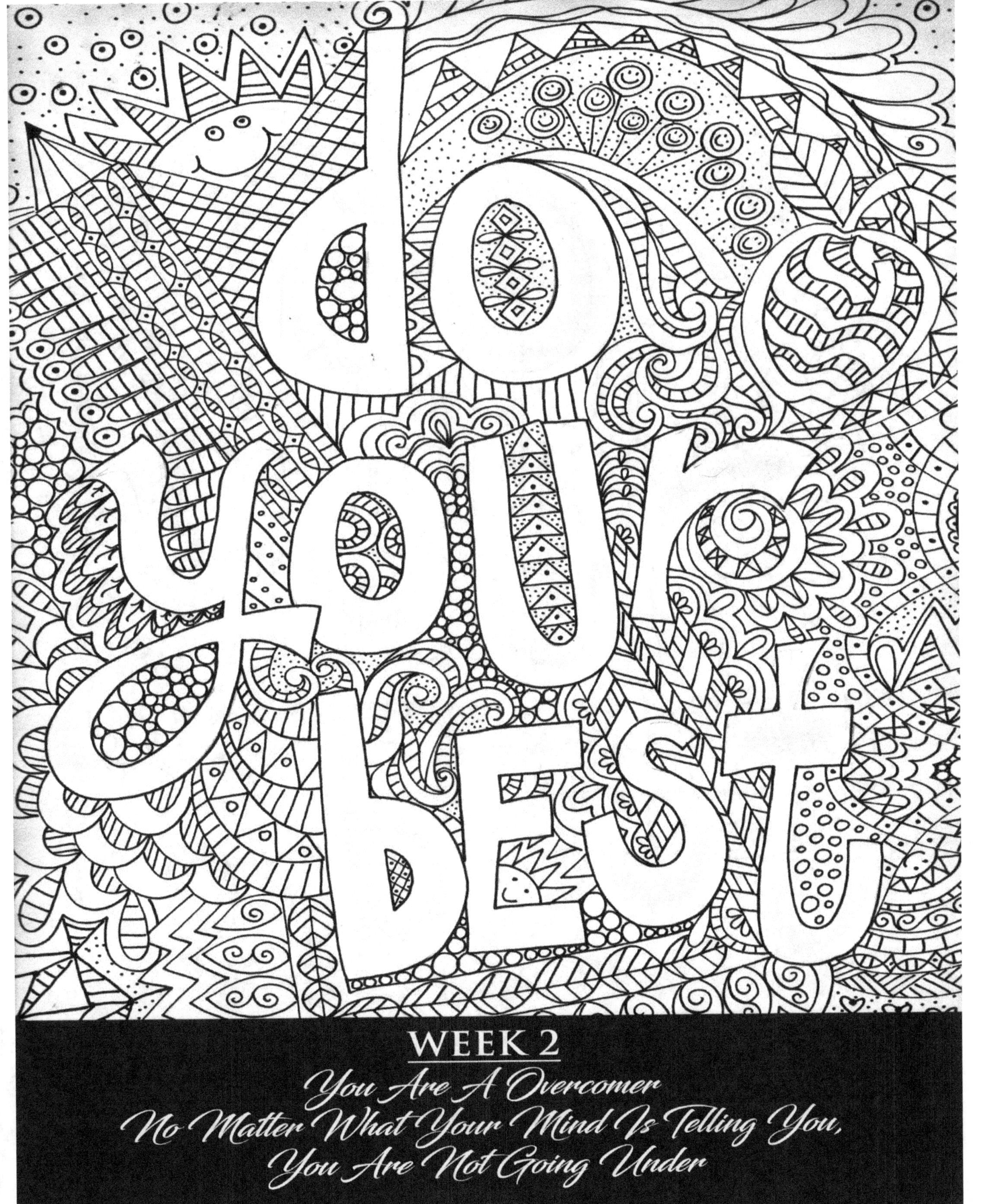

WEEK 2

You Are A Overcomer
No Matter What Your Mind Is Telling You,
You Are Not Going Under

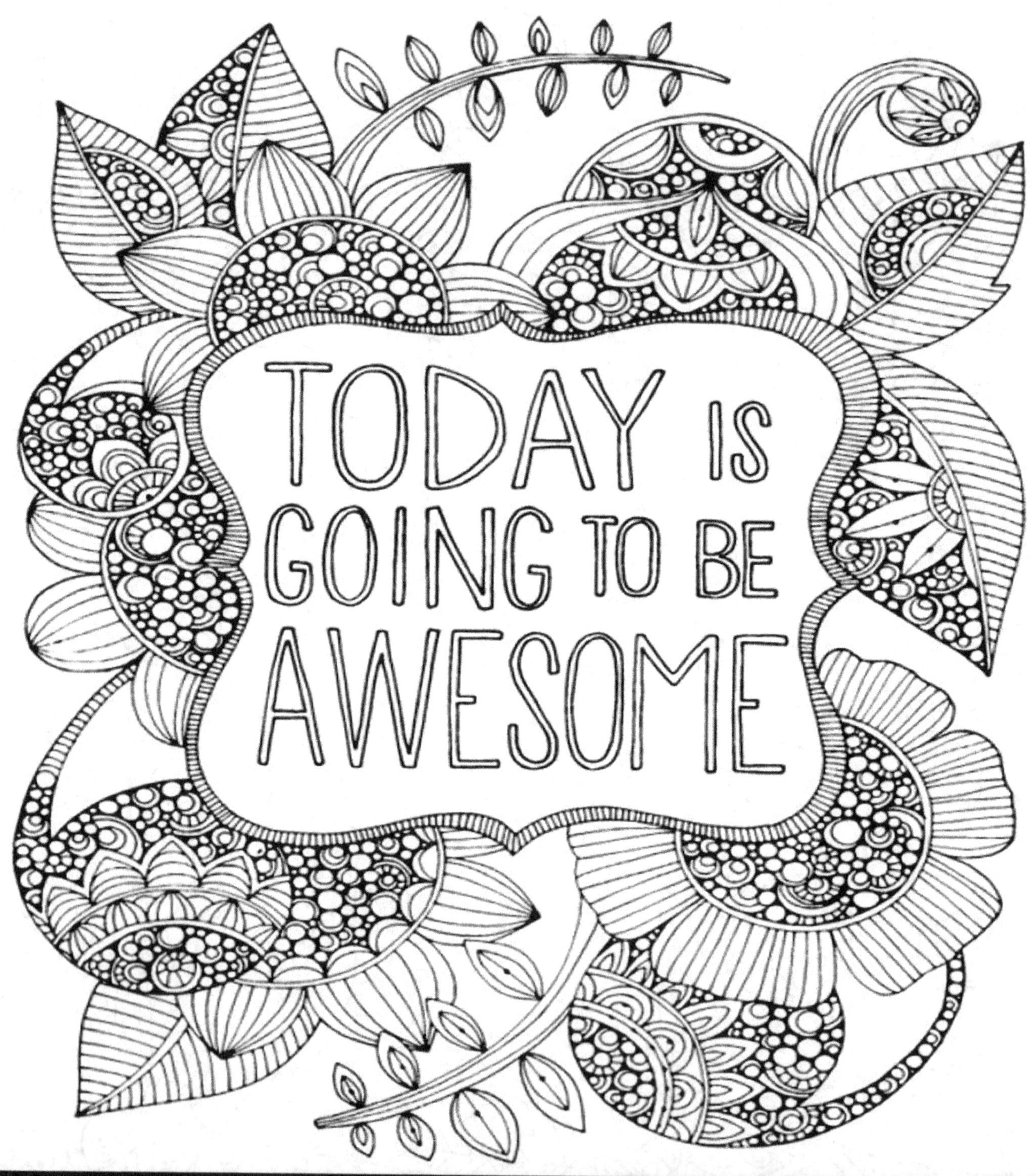

WEEK 3
Take Your Mental Wellness Journey One Day At A Time

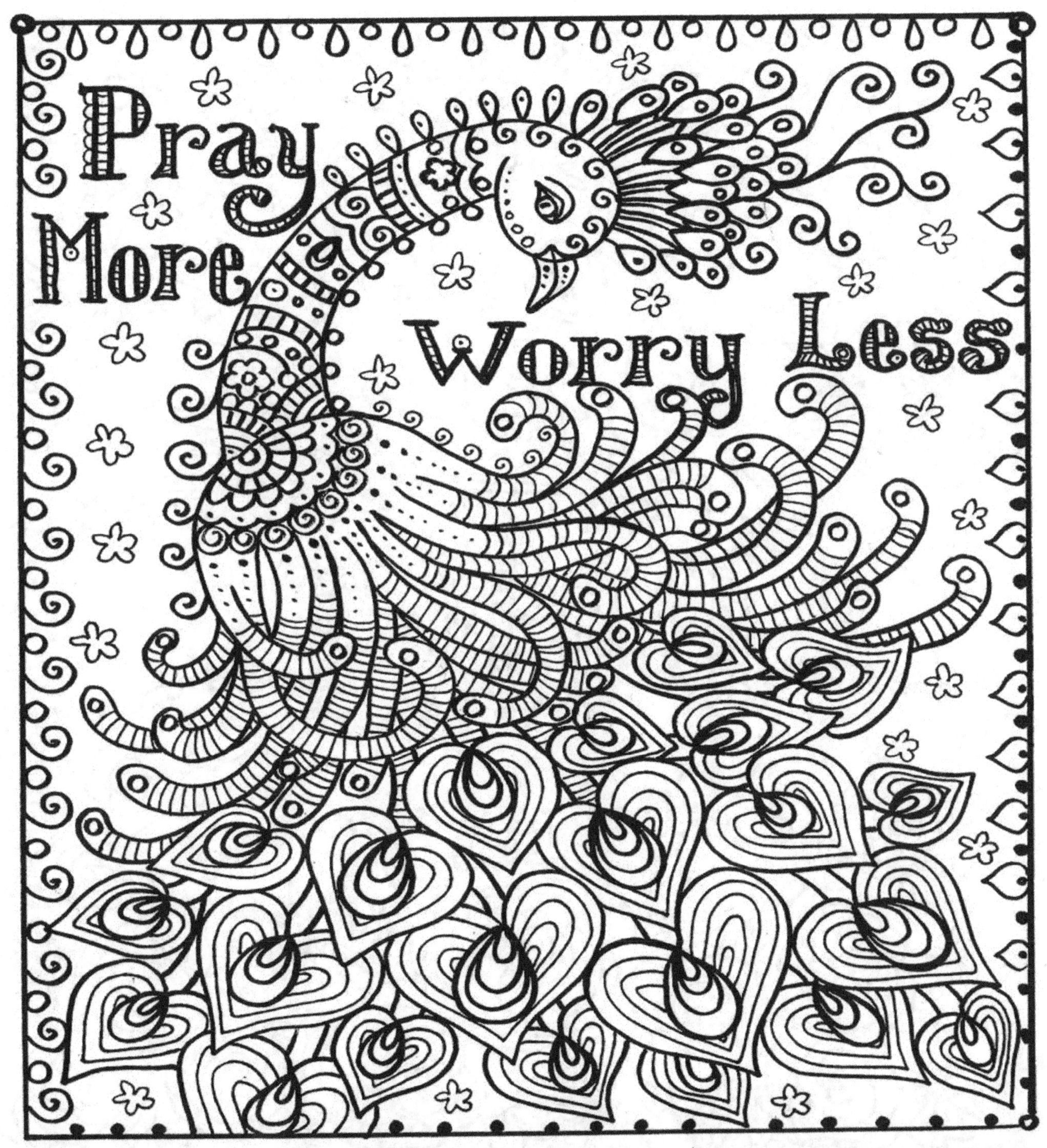

<u>WEEK 4</u>

Healing Does Not Take Place Over Night

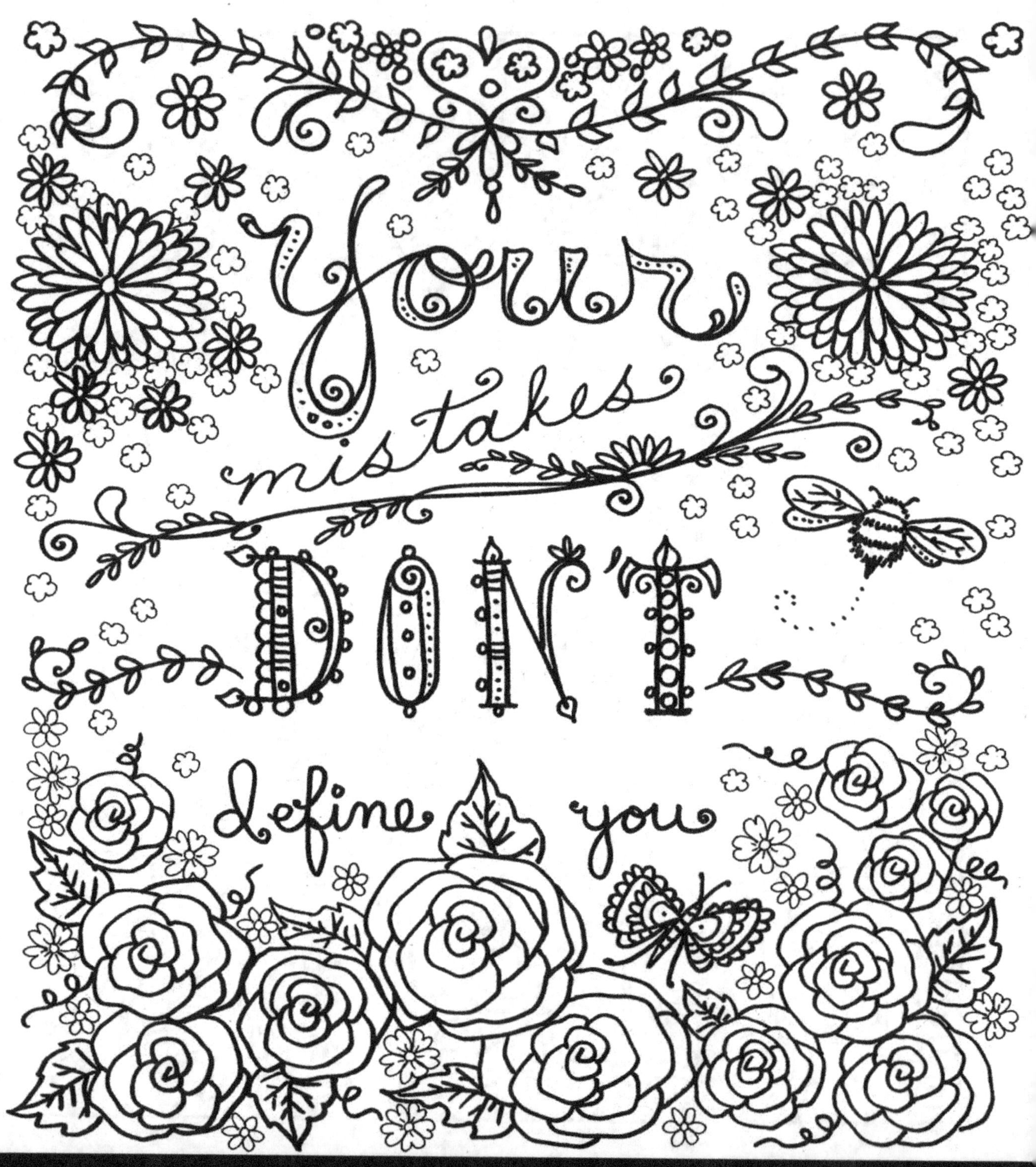

WEEK 5
Progress Is A Process

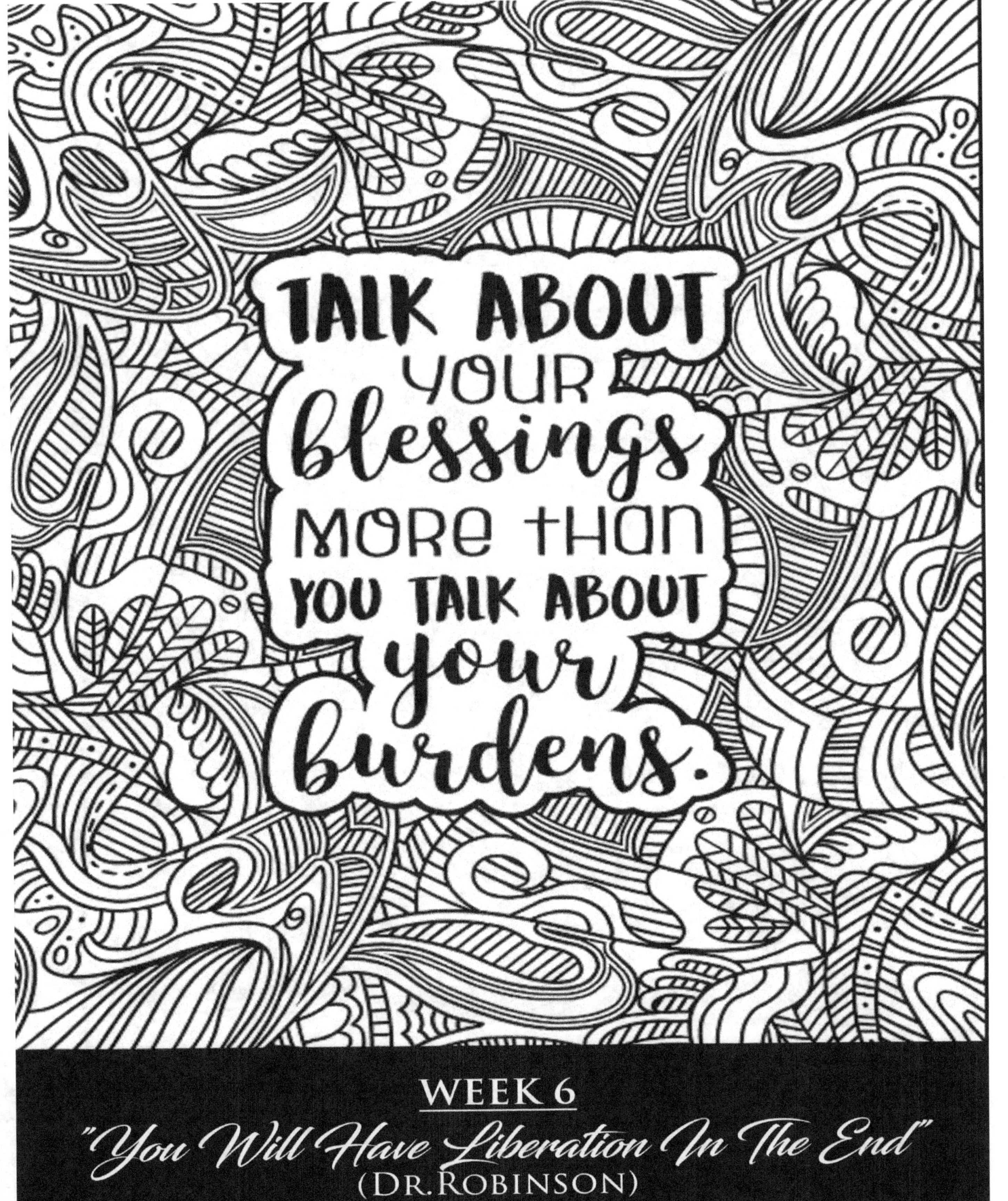

WEEK 6

"You Will Have Liberation In The End"
(DR. ROBINSON)

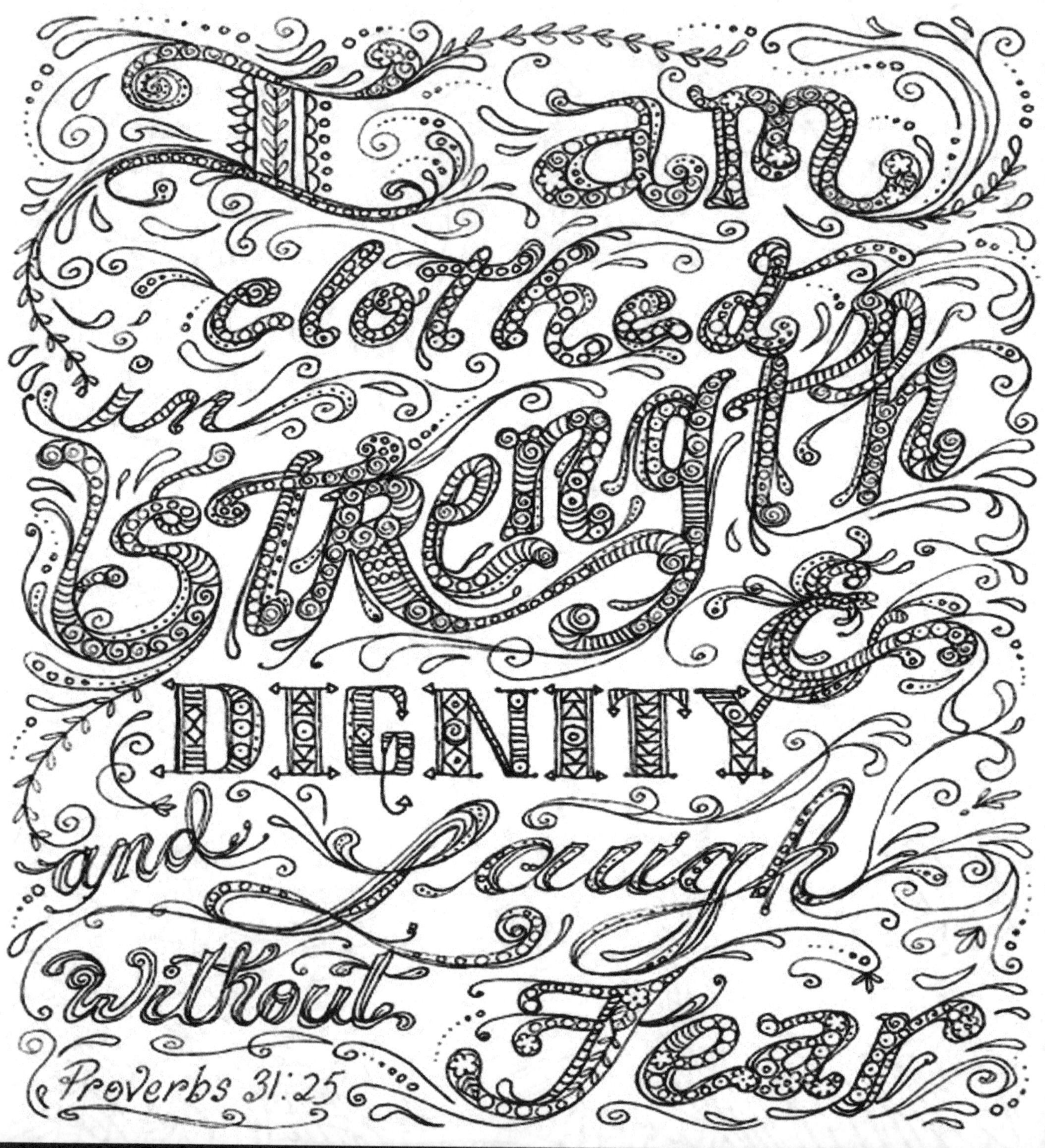

I am clothed in strength & DIGNITY and Laugh without Fear
Proverbs 31:25

WEEK 7
"You Have To Know, That You Know,
That You know, God Is Healing You" = Believe
DAD

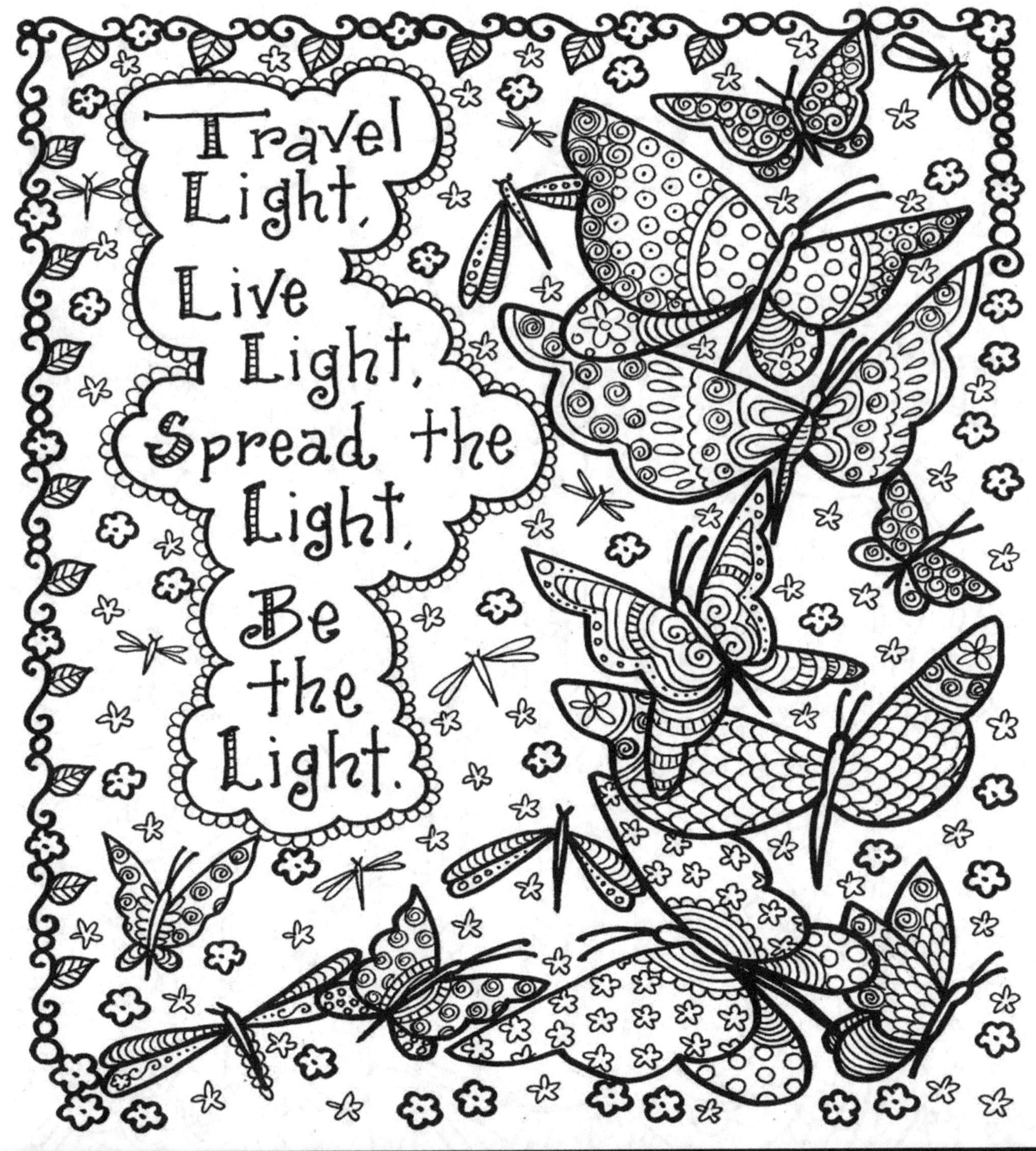

The Light Is Inside Of You

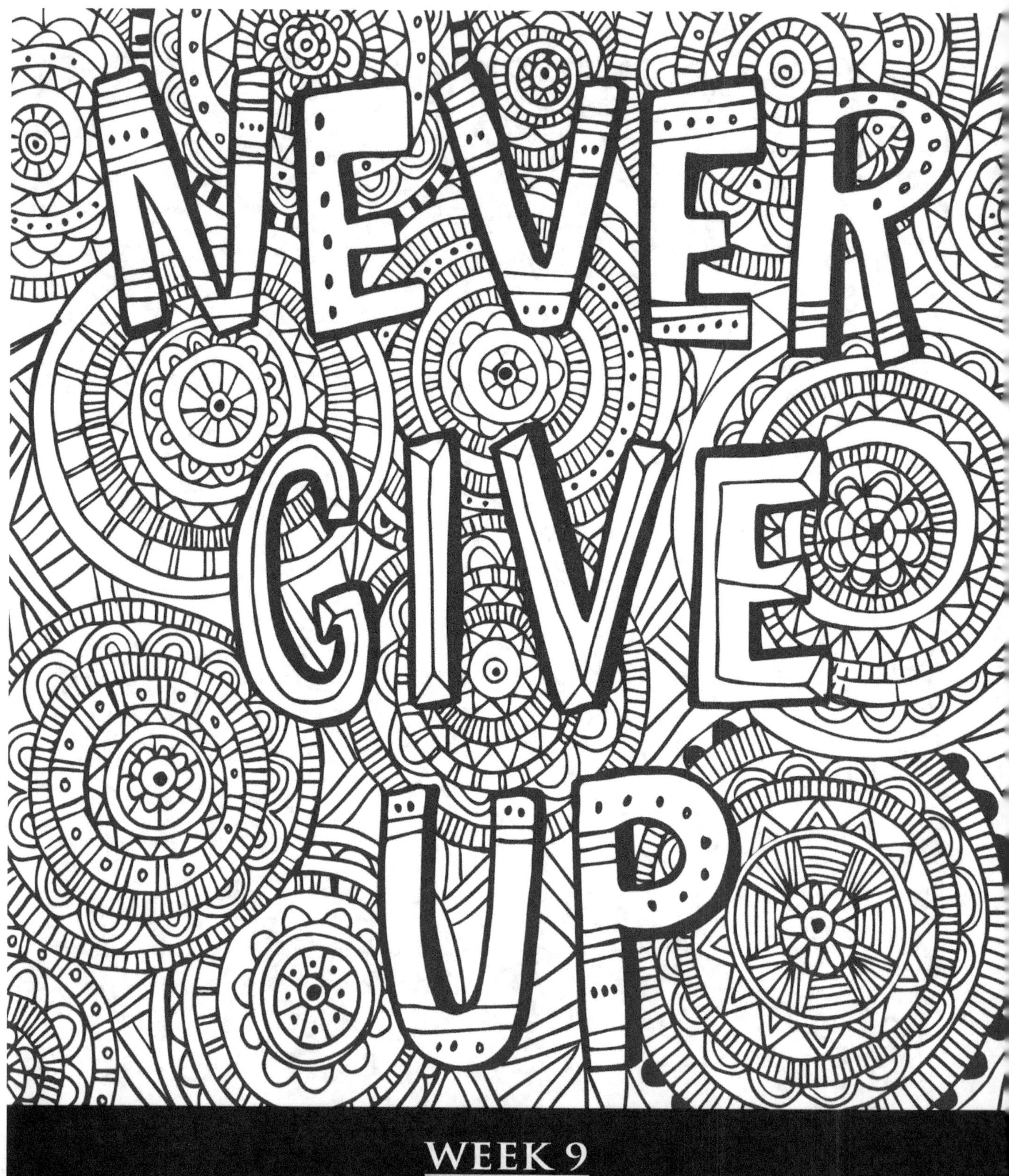

NEVER
GIVE
UP

WEEK 9
Keep Going

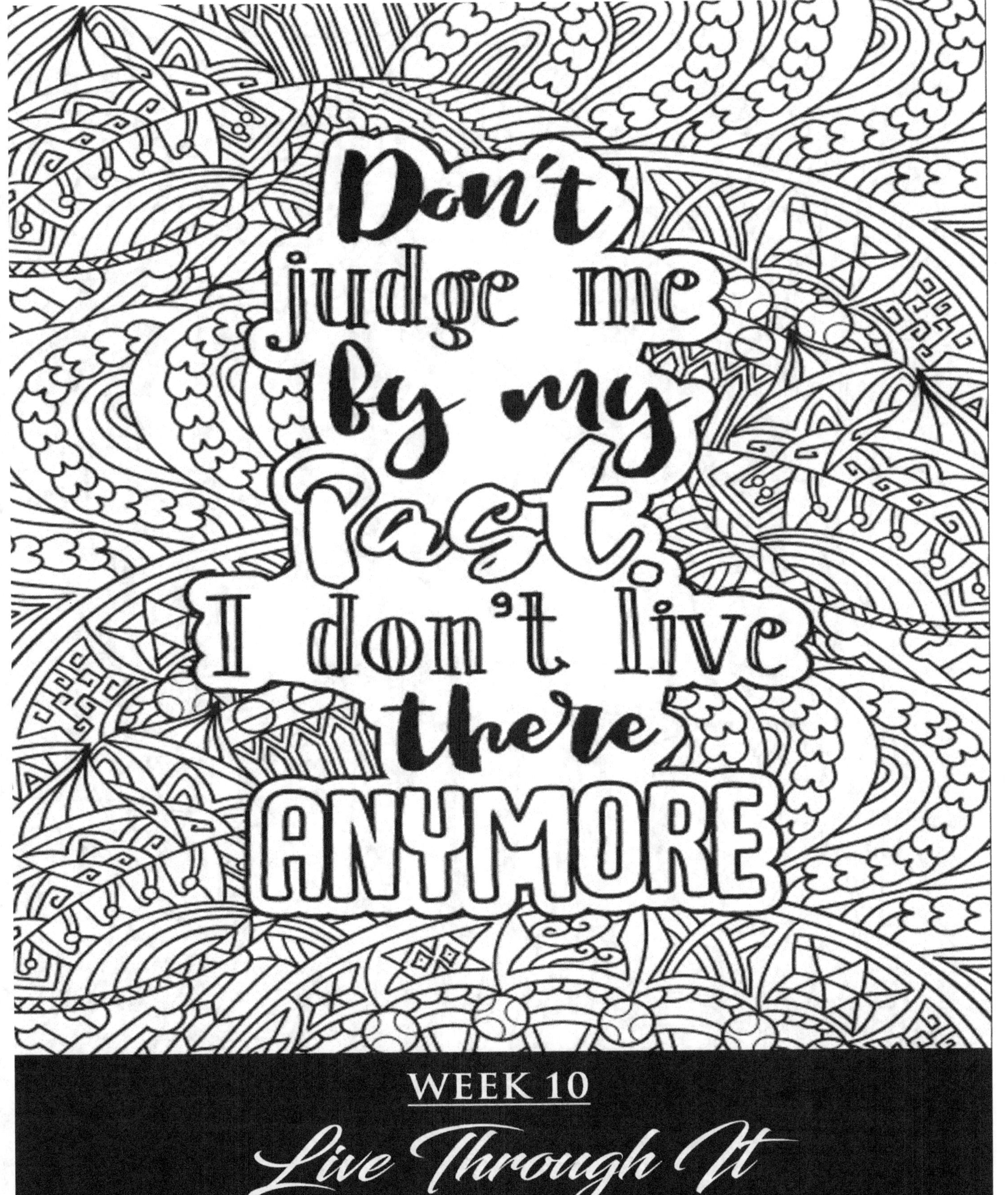

WEEK 10

Live Through It

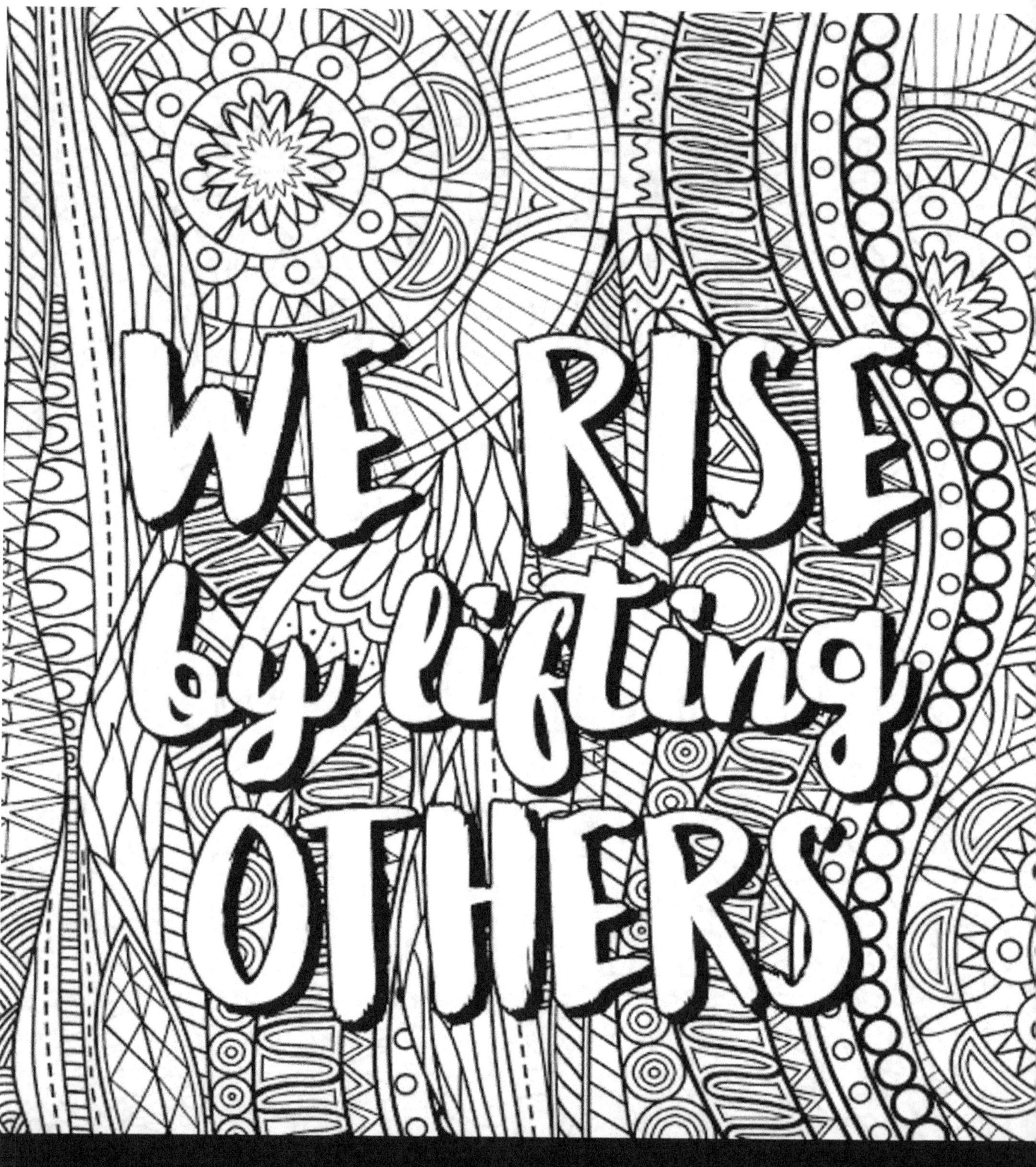

WE RISE
by lifting
OTHERS

WEEK 11
I Am Here With You

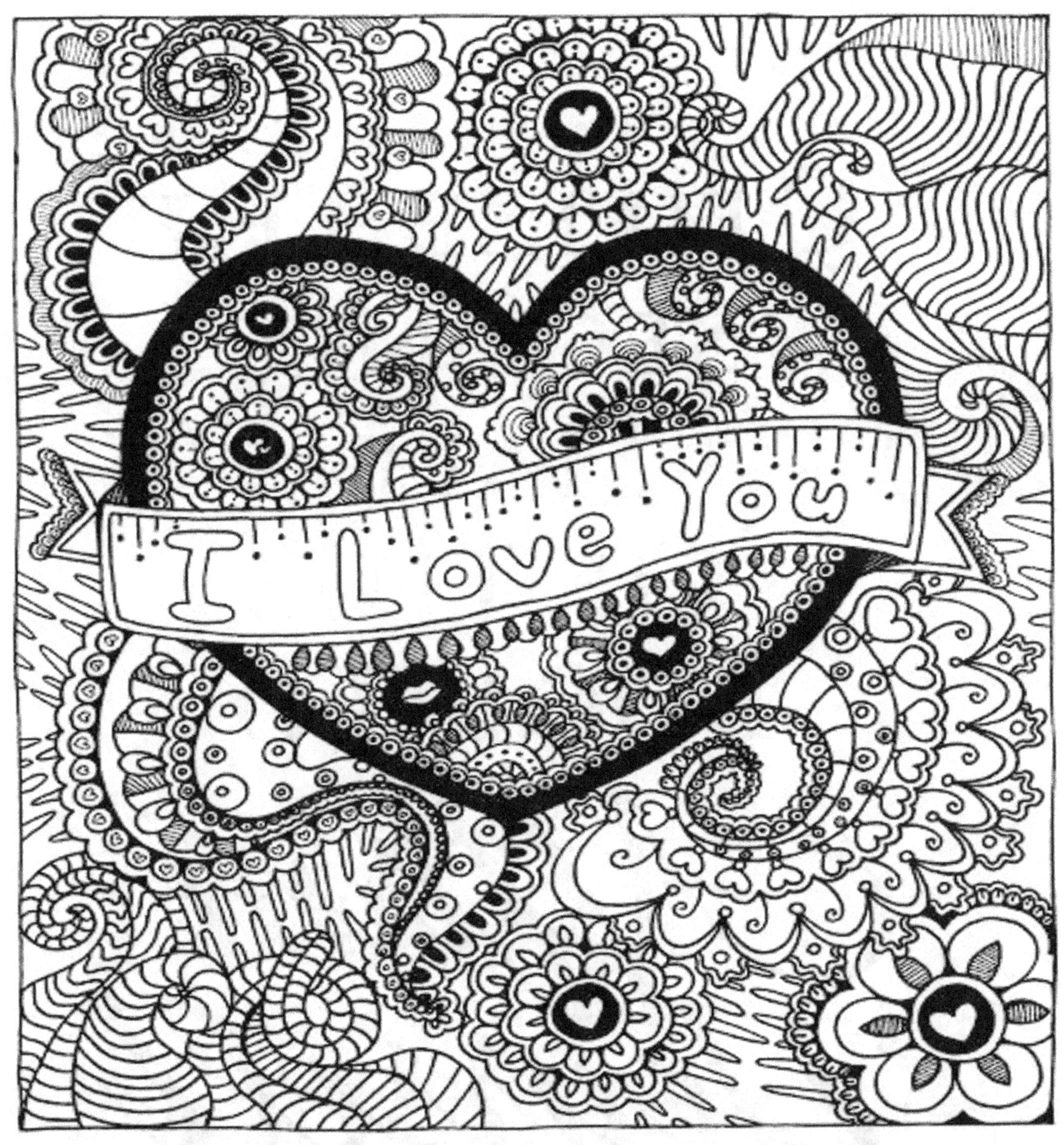

WEEK 12
I Love You
MOM

Utilize The Second Half Of This Book To

Affirm Yourself

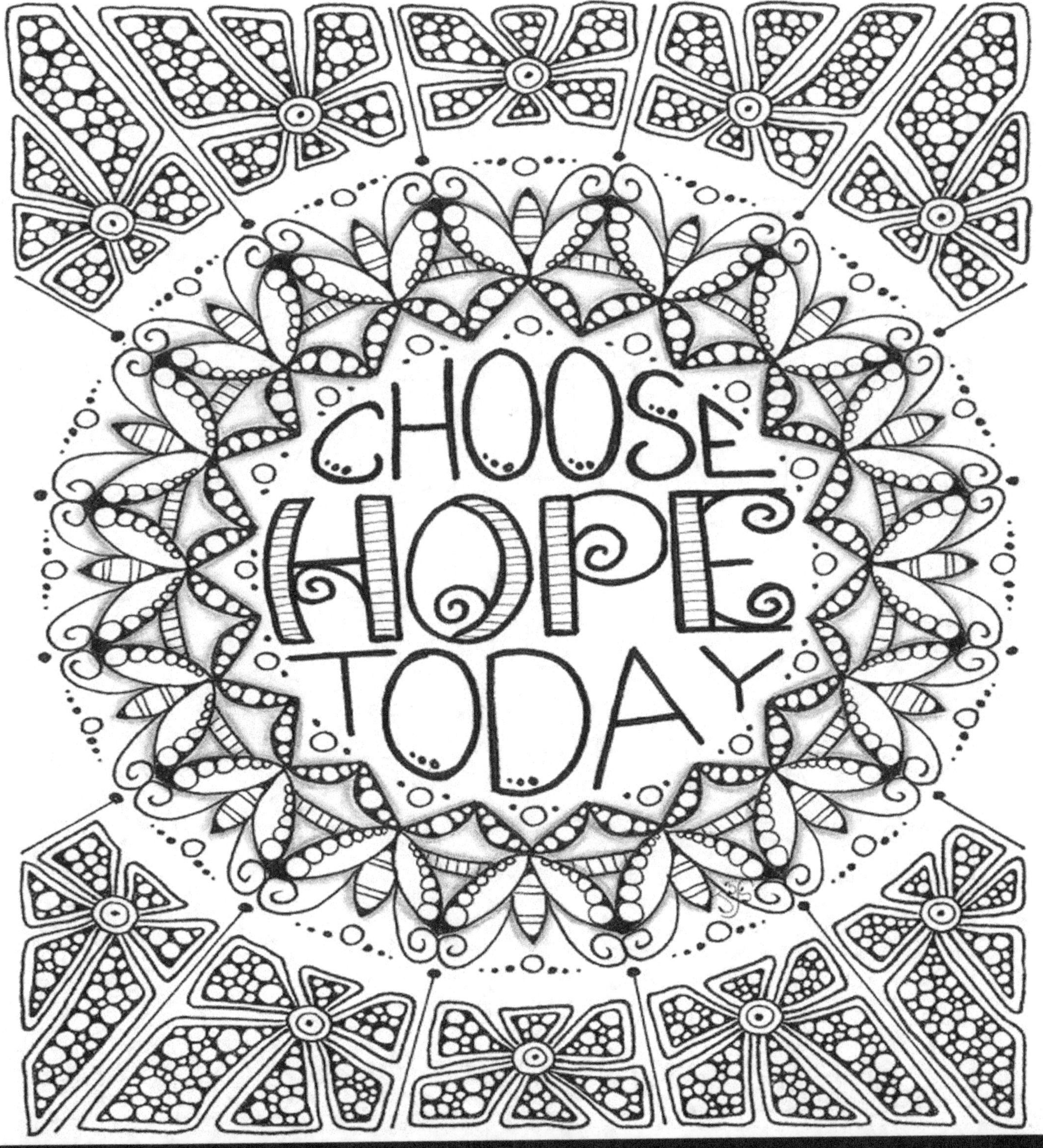

WEEK 13

I Can Win The Battle

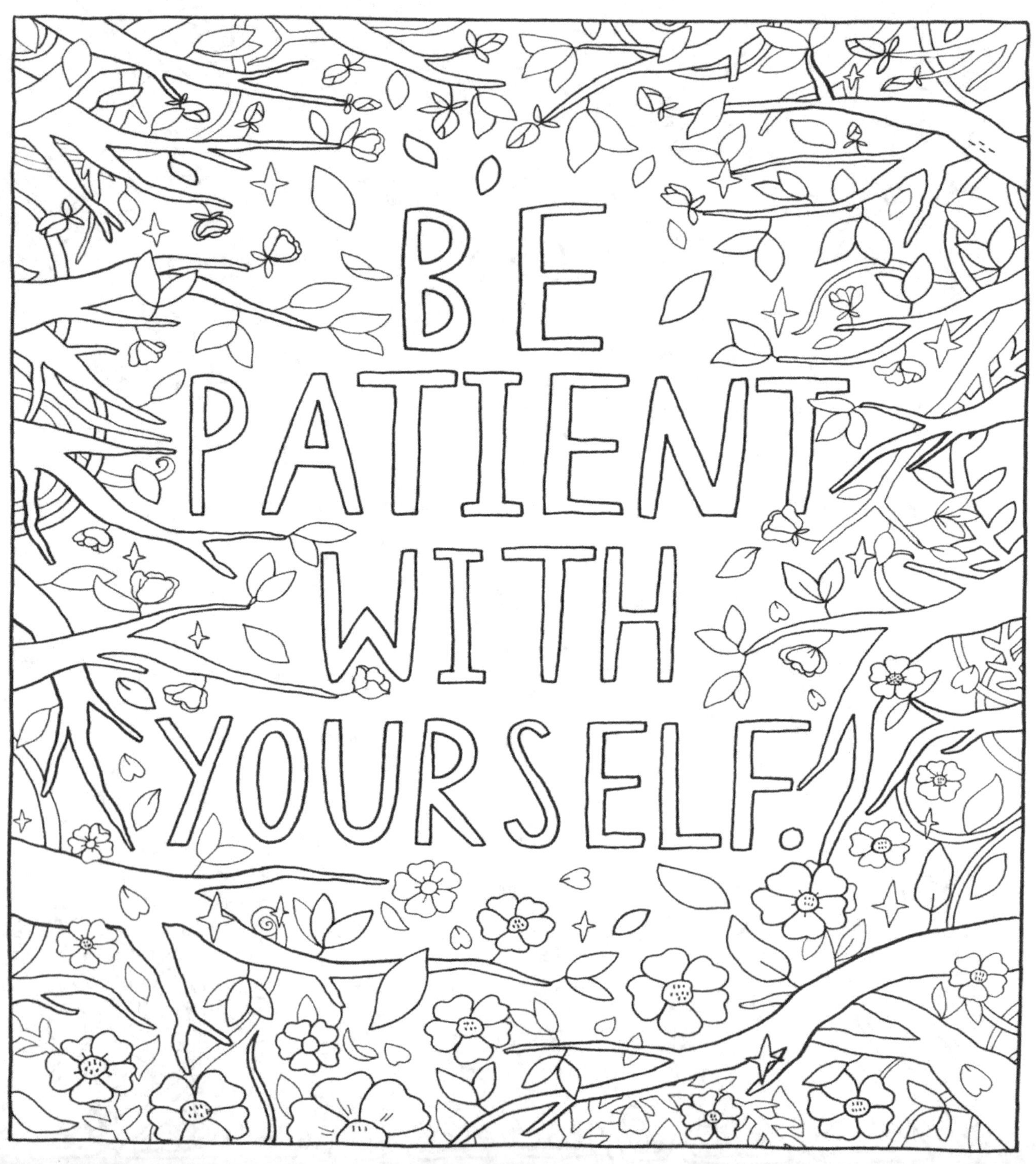

<u>**WEEK 14**</u>
Selfcare Comes First

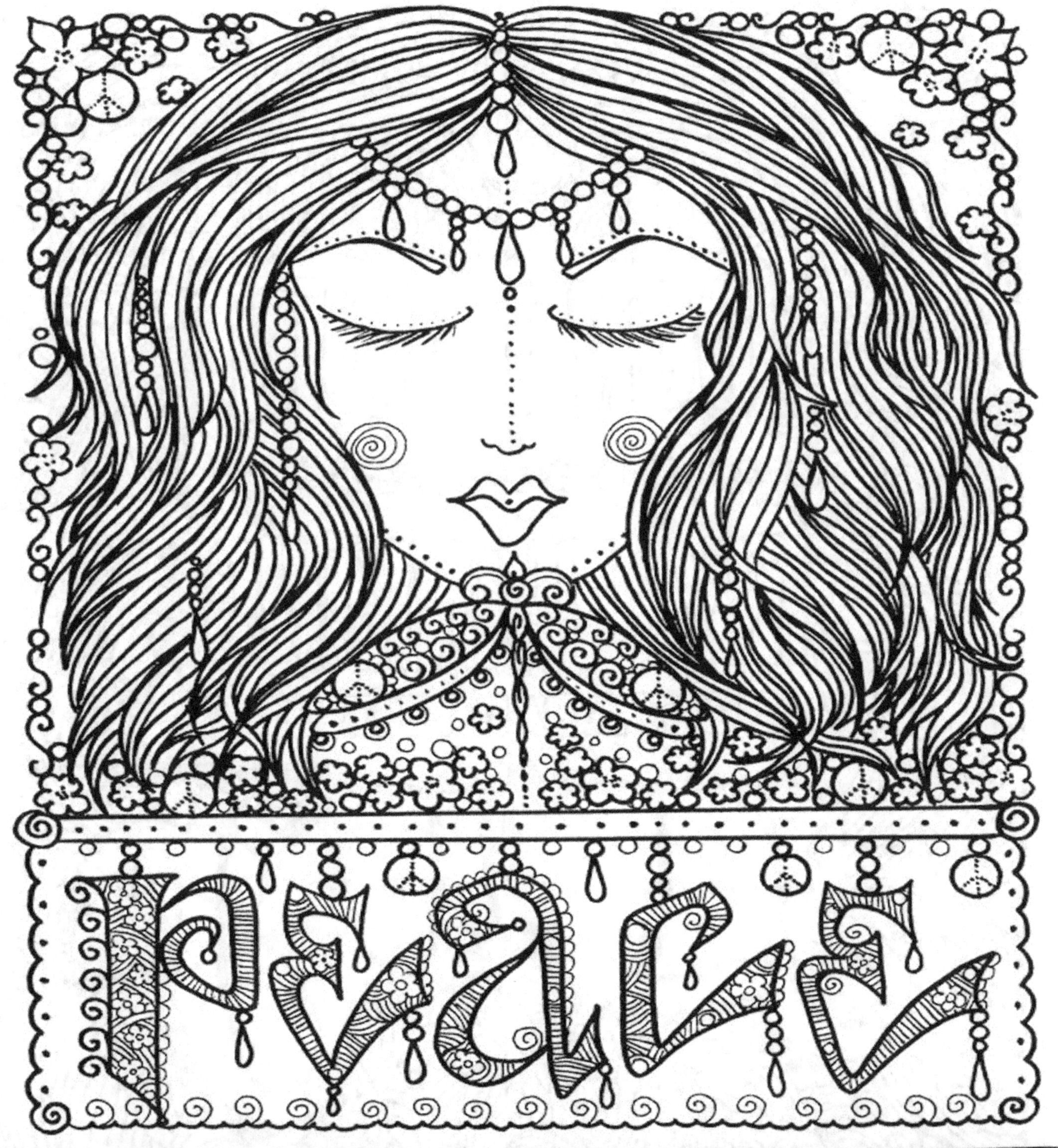

WEEK 15
I Will Get Rest

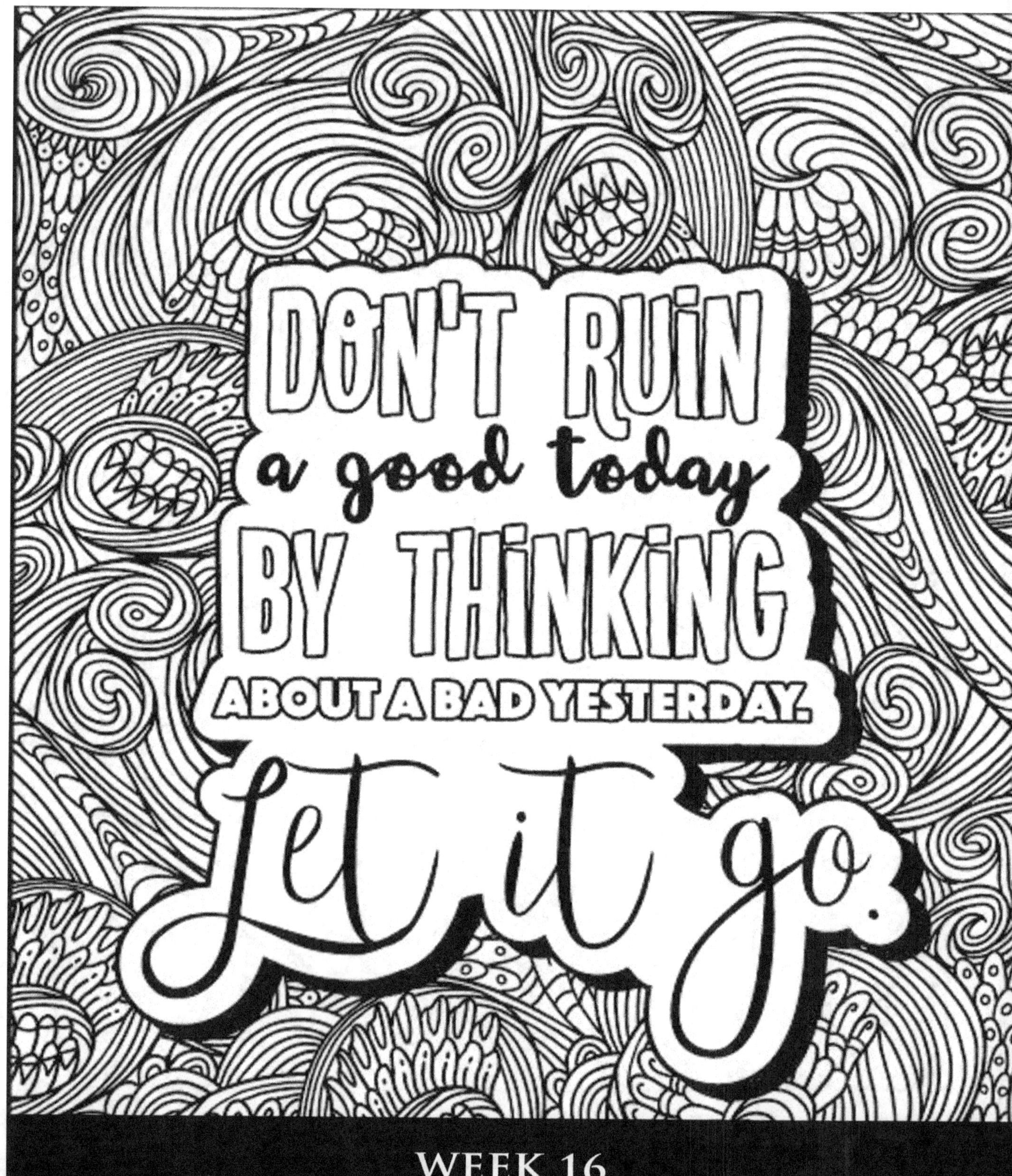

WEEK 16

I Will Not Give Up

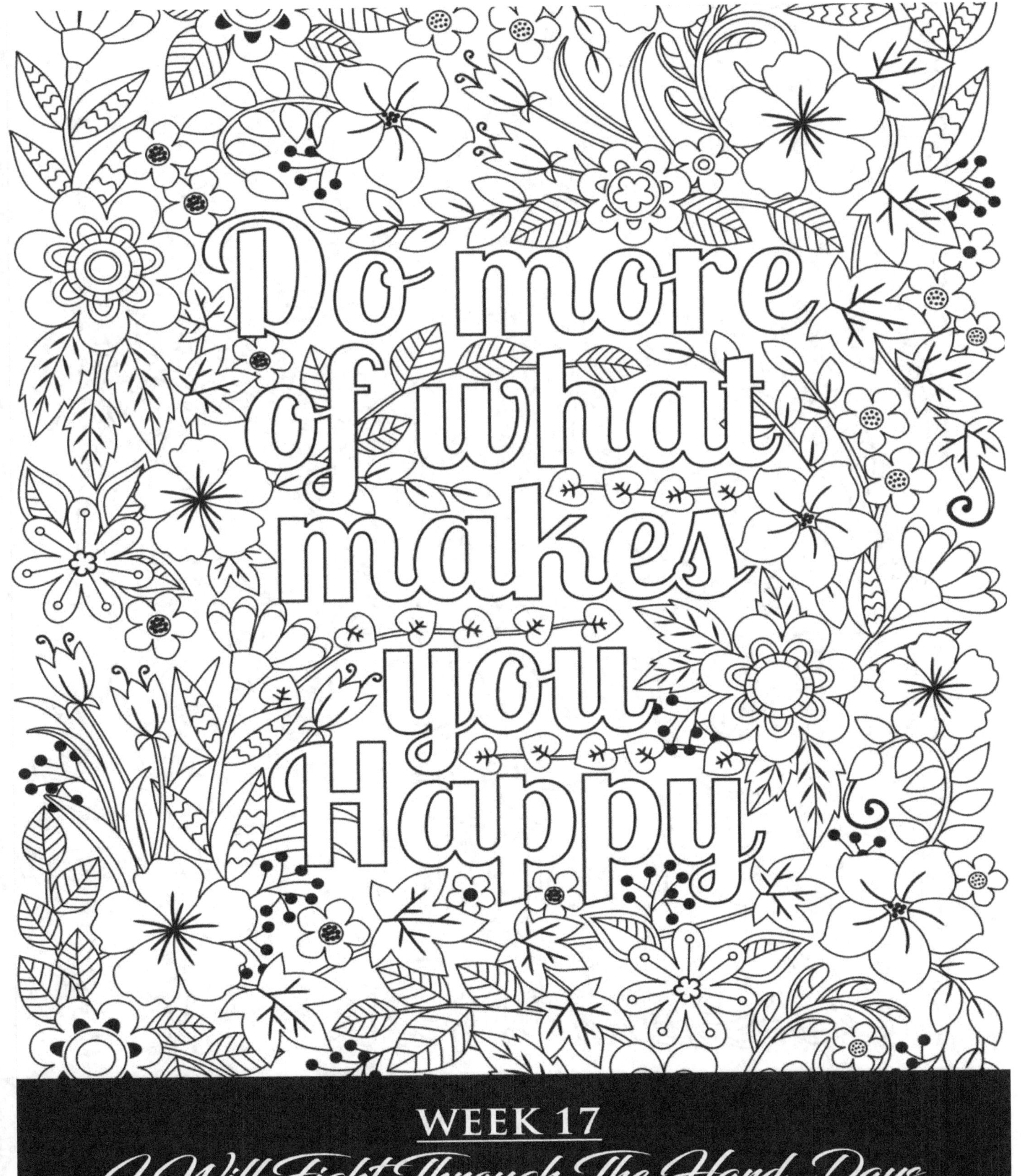

Do more of what makes you Happy

WEEK 17
I Will Fight Through The Hard Days

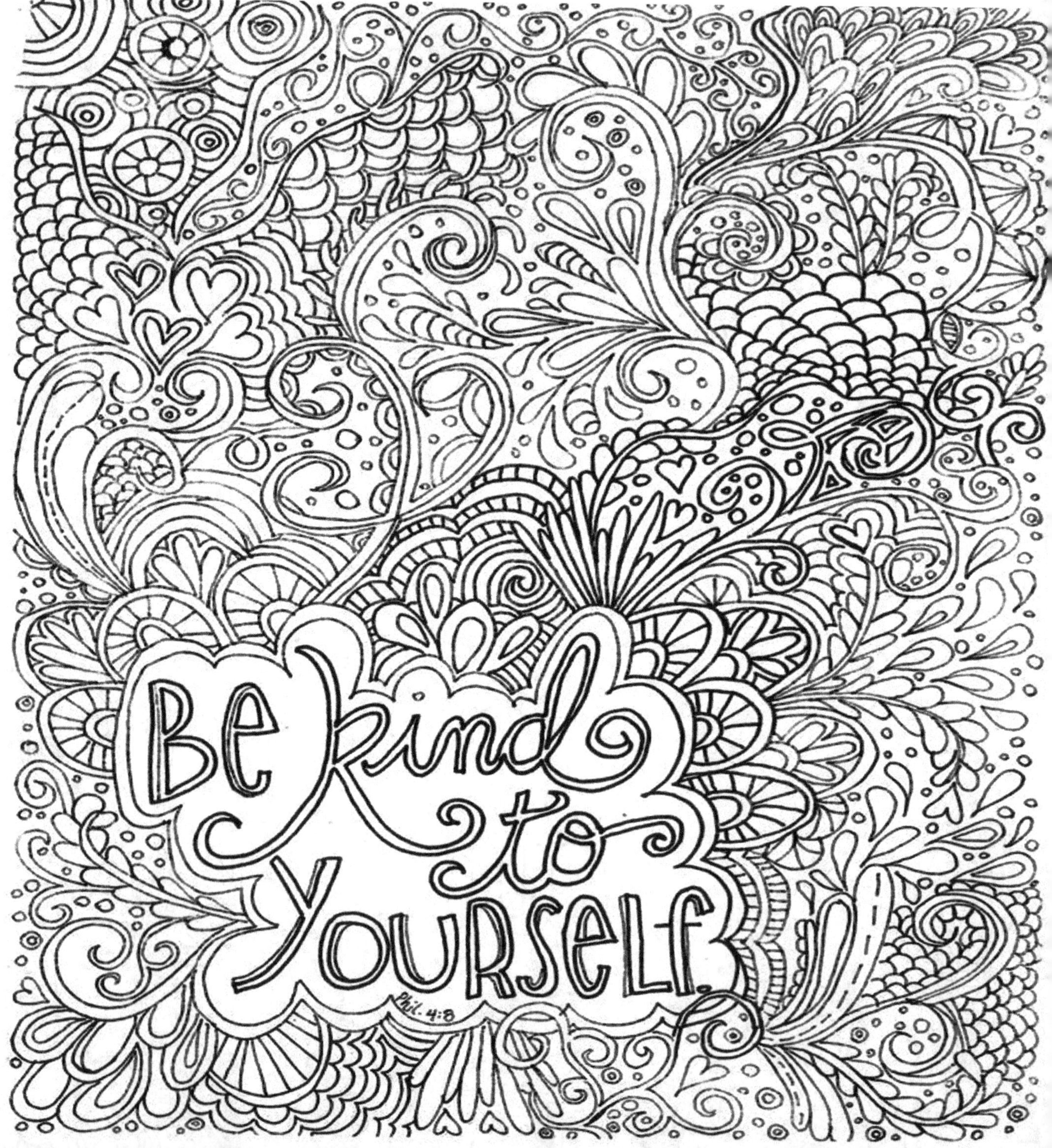

WEEK 18
I Can Pick Up The Broken Pieces

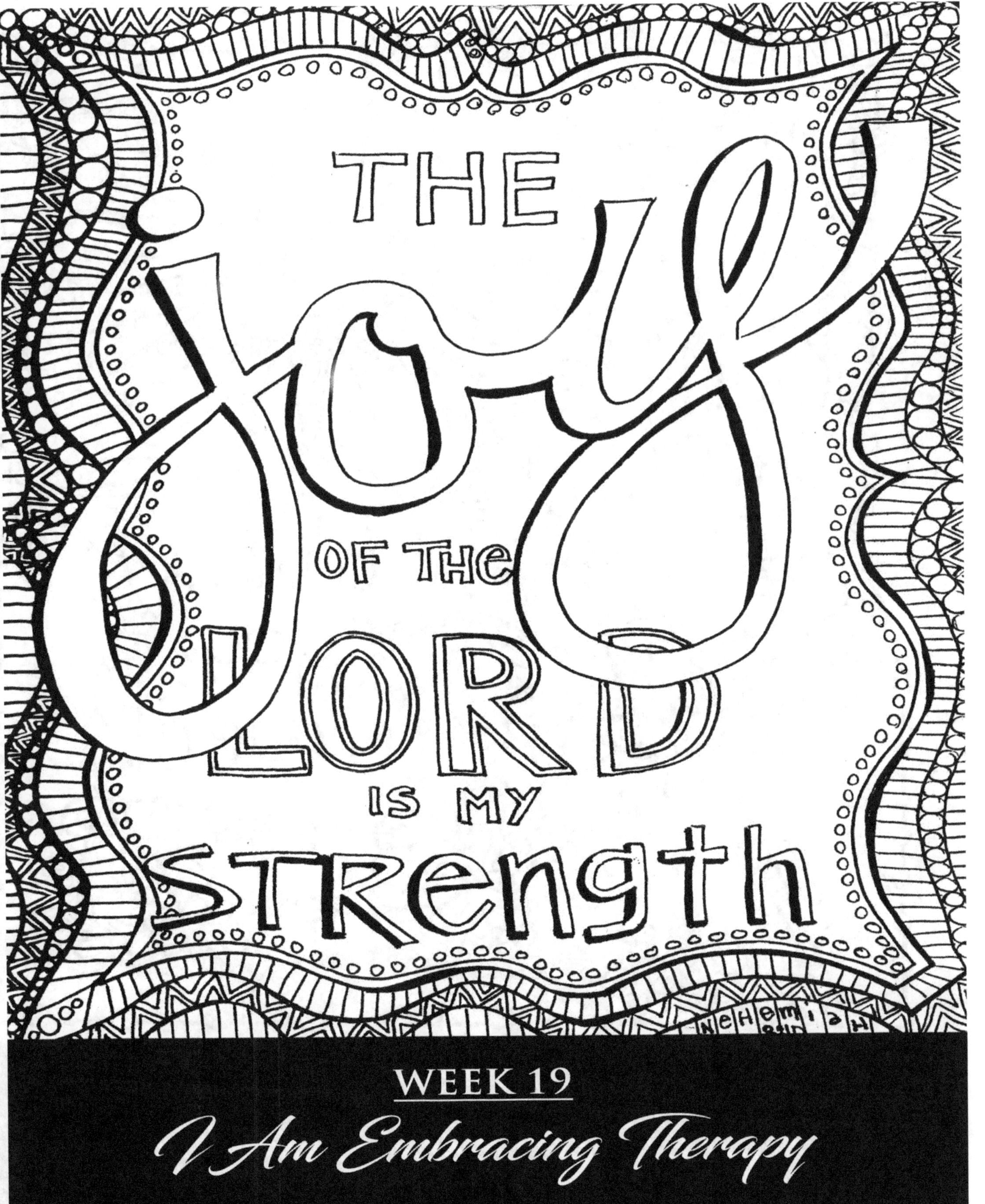

I Am Embracing Therapy

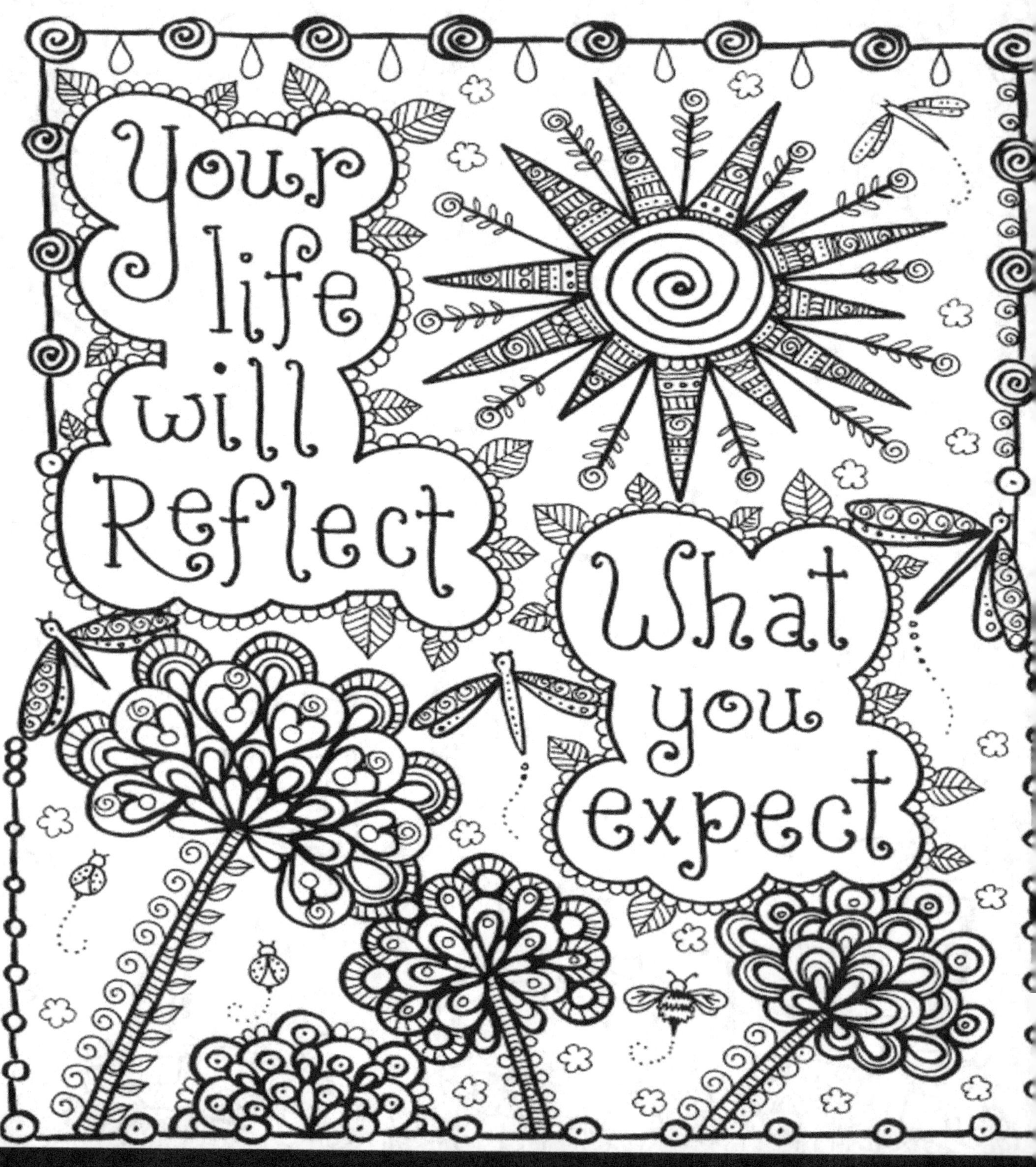

<u>WEEK 20</u>

Fear Does Not Control Me

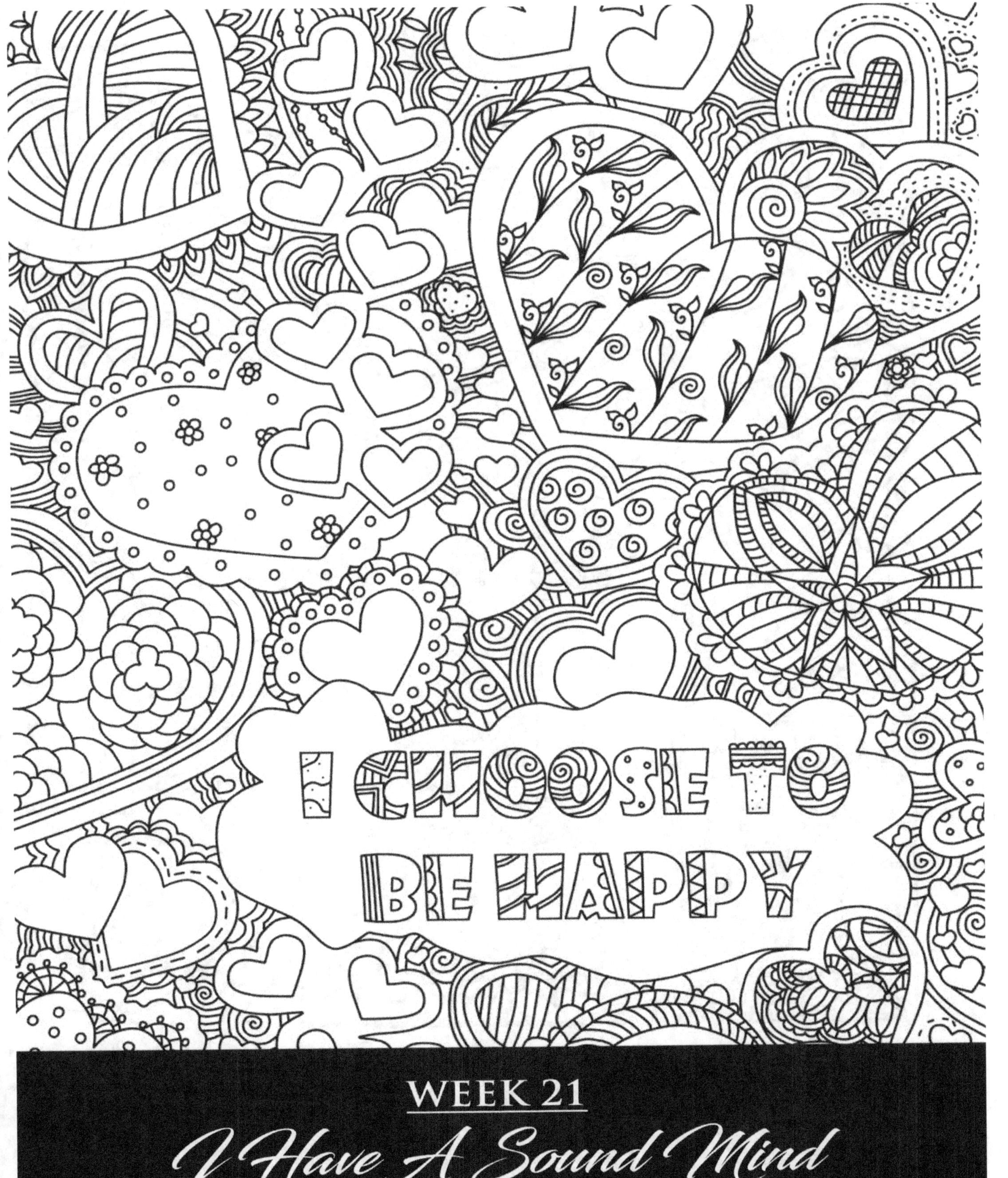

I CHOOSE TO BE HAPPY
WEEK 21
I Have A Sound Mind

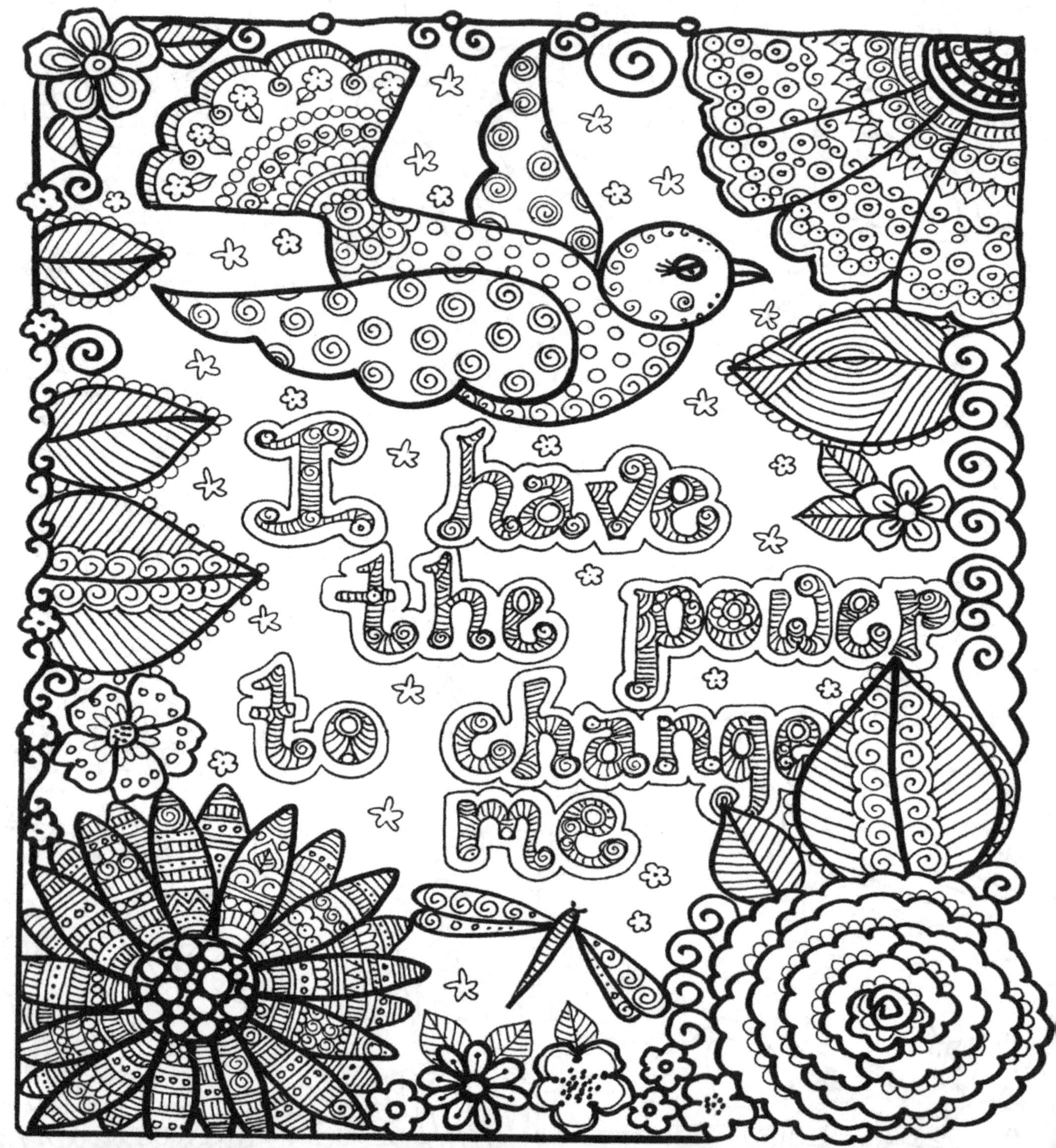

I have the power to change me

WEEK 22
I Will Work towards the
Best Version Of Me

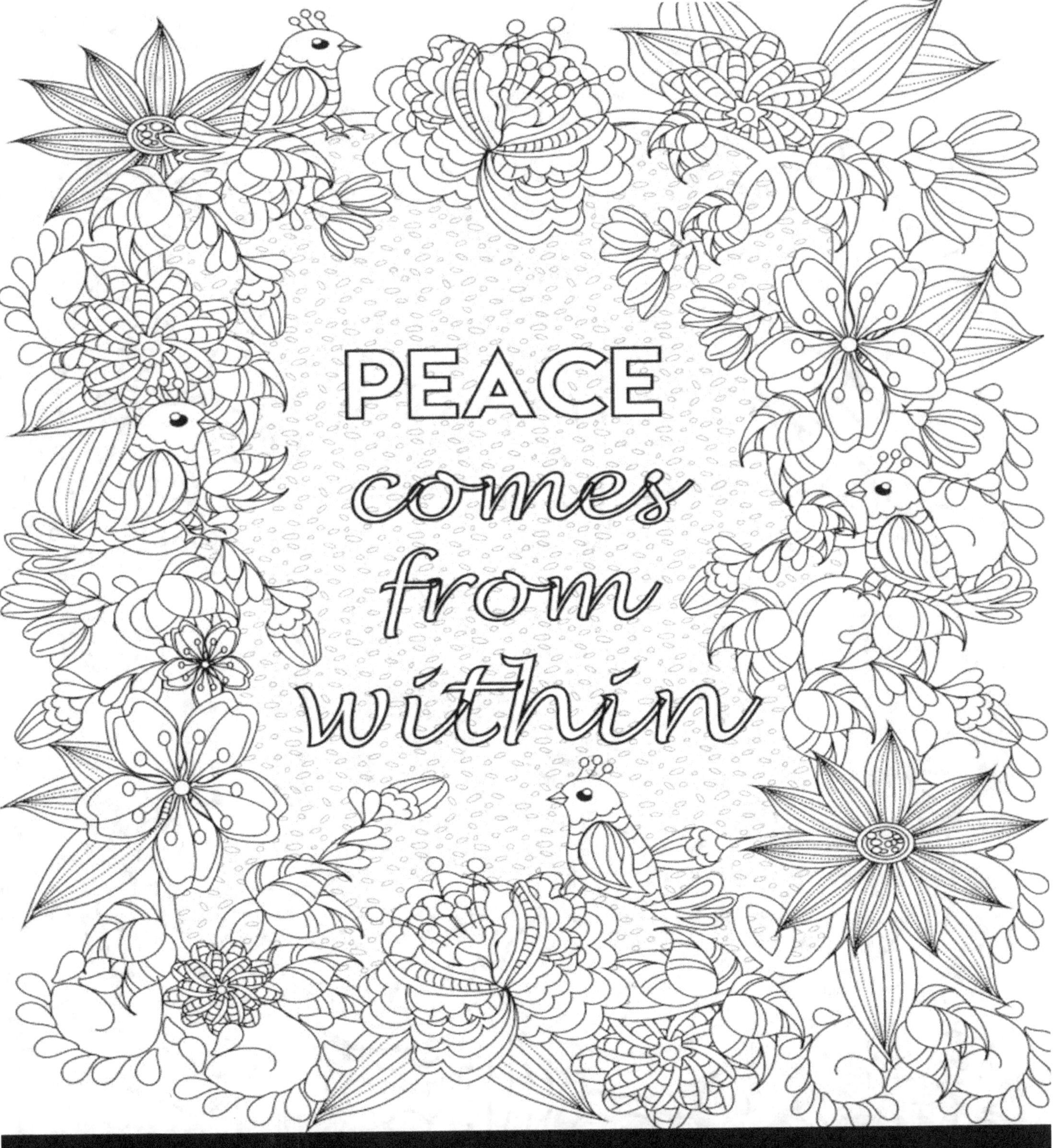

PEACE
comes
from
within

WEEK 23
Mental Wellness Is Key

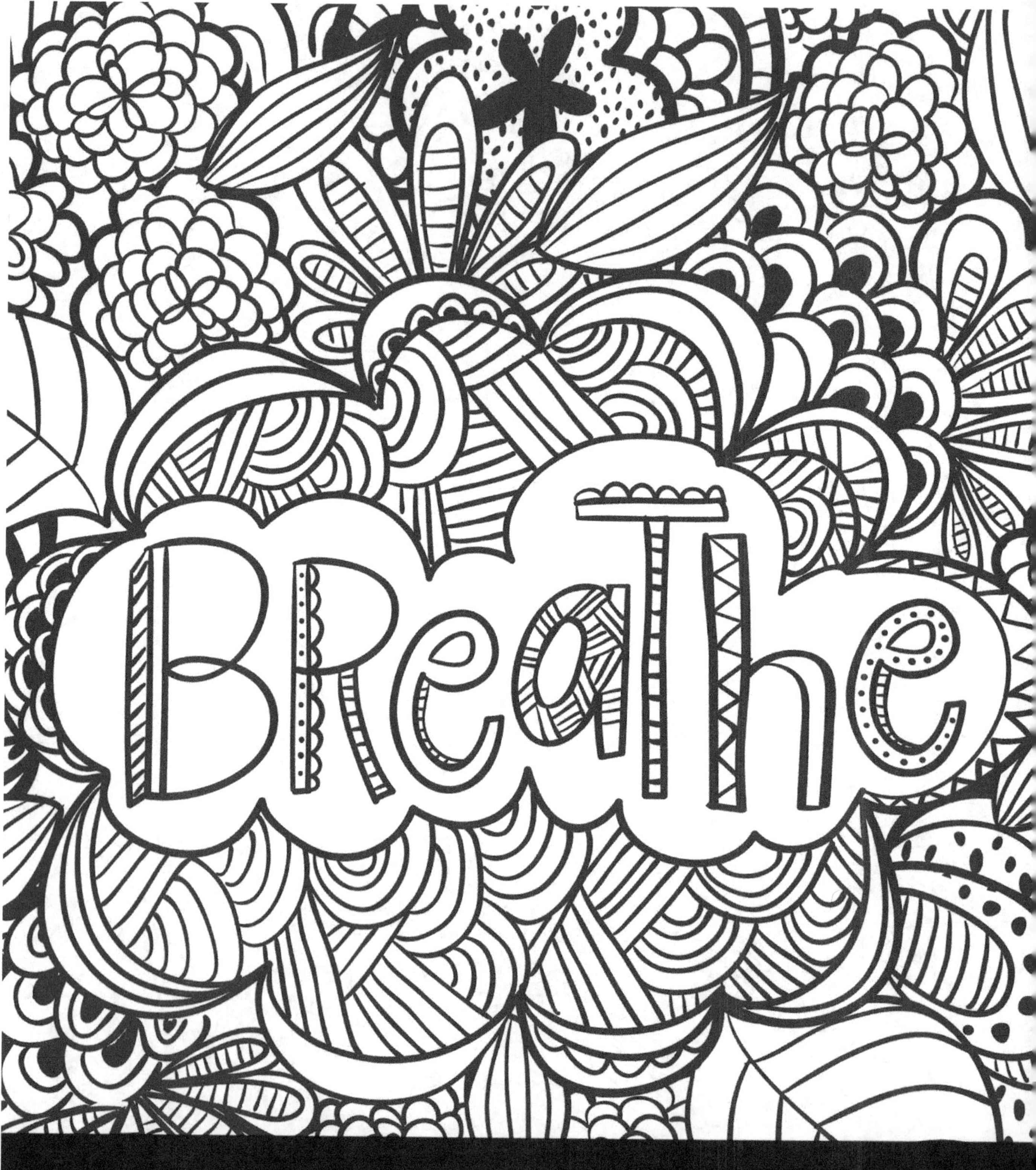

BReaThe

WEEK 24
I Feel Free